ANTI-INFLAMMATORY DIET MEAL PREP:

Tips, Recipes, and Strategies for Success

Richard S. Daniels

Table of Contents:

Chapter 1:

Introduction to the Anti-Inflammatory Diet

Anti-Inflammatory diet has gained popularity in recent years due to its numerous health benefits, including reducing chronic inflammation, which is linked to many chronic diseases such as heart disease, diabetes, and cancer. This chapter will provide readers with an overview of the Anti-Inflammatory diet and its benefits.

What is an Anti-Inflammatory diet?

A diet in the conventional sense is not what an anti-inflammatory diet is. Instead, it refers to a manner of eating that places an emphasis on full, nutrient-dense foods and reduces or completely avoids processed and inflammatory foods. The foundation of the anti-inflammatory diet is the idea that specific foods can either increase or decrease inflammation in the body. By making anti-inflammatory food choices, we can lower our chance of developing chronic diseases and improve our general health and well-being.

What are the benefits of an Anti-Inflammatory diet?

The Anti-Inflammatory diet has been shown to have numerous health benefits, including:

- Reduced Risk of Chronic Diseases: Numerous chronic diseases, including cancer, diabetes, and heart disease, are associated with chronic inflammation. We can lower the risk of these diseases by eating an anti-inflammatory diet and lowering inflammation.

- Improved Digestive Health: Many meals high in anti-inflammatory compounds can also lead to digestive problems like gas, bloating, and constipation. We can enhance digestive health by limiting certain items and consuming anti-inflammatory foods instead.

- Weight Management: Whole, nutritious foods that are naturally low in calories are prioritized by the anti-inflammatory diet. This may help you regulate your weight and keep it at a healthy level.

- Improved Mood: Depression and anxiety have been linked to chronic inflammation. An anti-inflammatory diet can help us lower inflammation, which can enhance our overall health and well-being.

What foods are included in the Anti-Inflammatory diet?

The anti-inflammatory diet emphasizes whole, nutrient-dense foods, such as

- Fruits and vegetables
- Whole grains
- Nuts and seeds
- Legumes
- Fatty fish (such as salmon)
- Healthy fats (such as olive oil and avocado)

Foods that are limited or avoided in the anti-inflammatory diet include:

- Processed foods
- Sugar and refined carbohydrates
- Red meat and processed meats
- Fried foods
- Trans fats

A diet that prioritizes whole, nutrient-dense meals and restricts or completely avoids processed, inflammatory foods is known as an anti-inflammatory diet. We can lower chronic inflammation and enhance our general health and well-being by consuming anti-inflammatory foods. The reader will find useful tips and recipes for adopting the anti-inflammatory diet into their daily lives in the chapters that follow.

Chapter 2:

The Science Behind Inflammation

What is inflammation?

Inflammation is the body's natural response to injury or infection. When a part of the body is injured or infected, the immune system responds by releasing white blood cells, which produce inflammation. Inflammation is necessary to heal the body and fight off infections.

Acute inflammation is a transient reaction that develops in the body in response to injury or infection. It exhibits discomfort, heat, swelling, and redness. Acute inflammation, which typically lasts a few days, is essential for recovery.

On the other hand, chronic inflammation is a long-lasting reaction that develops when the immune system is continuously engaged. Numerous chronic diseases can develop from chronic inflammation, which can harm healthy tissue.

How does chronic inflammation affect the body?

Chronic inflammation has been linked to many chronic diseases, including:

- Heart Disease: Chronic inflammation increases the risk of heart disease by damaging the blood vessel lining and causing atherosclerosis, a condition in which plaque builds up in the arteries.

- Diabetes: Insulin resistance, a disease in which the body's cells do not respond to insulin as intended, can cause chronic inflammation and raise the risk of developing diabetes.

- Cancer: Chronic inflammation can damage DNA and increase the risk of cancer.

- Alzheimer's Disease: Chronic inflammation can damage brain cells and increase the risk of Alzheimer's disease.

Factors That Contribute to Chronic Inflammation

Several factors can contribute to chronic inflammation, including:

- Poor diet: Consuming a lot of processed foods, sweets, and bad fats might increase inflammation in the body.

- Lack of Exercise: Regular exercise can help treat chronic inflammation by lowering the body's synthesis of inflammatory chemicals.

- Stress: The body may produce inflammatory chemicals as a result of ongoing stress.

- Environmental Toxins: Chronic inflammation can be exacerbated by environmental pollutants, such as pollution and chemicals.

- Genetics: A genetic tendency to chronic inflammation may exist in some individuals, which may raise their risk of chronic illness development.

Strategies for Reducing Chronic Inflammation:

The good news is that several strategies can help reduce chronic inflammation, including:

- Eating an Anti-Inflammatory Diet: A diet low in processed foods and high in whole, nutrient-dense foods is known as an "anti-inflammatory diet." Fruits, vegetables, whole grains, lean meats, and healthy fats are some examples of these foods.

- Exercise regularly: Regular exercise can help treat chronic inflammation by lowering the body's synthesis of inflammatory chemicals.

- Managing Stress: Deep breathing, yoga, meditation, and other stress-reduction practices can help lessen chronic inflammation.

- Reducing Exposure to Environmental Toxins: Chronic inflammation can be lessened by limiting exposure to environmental pollutants such as pollution and chemicals.

- Getting Enough Sleep: Getting enough sleep is important for reducing chronic inflammation and promoting overall health.

When the immune system is continually engaged, chronic inflammation develops as a long-term reaction. Numerous chronic diseases can develop from chronic inflammation, which can harm healthy tissue. Chronic inflammation can be caused by a variety of factors, including a poor diet, inactivity, stress, pollutants in the environment, and heredity. It is feasible to minimize chronic inflammation and enhance general health by changing one's lifestyle by adopting anti-inflammatory dietary habits, exercising frequently, managing stress, minimizing exposure to environmental contaminants, and getting enough sleep.

The Immune System and Inflammation

The immune system is in charge of defending the body against external threats like viruses, bacteria, and other dangerous diseases. The immune system reacts to a foreign intruder entering the body by releasing white blood cells to combat and eliminate the invader.

An important aspect of the immune system's reaction to outside invaders is inflammation. An inflammatory response is brought on by the release of white blood cells and aids in isolating and eliminating the foreign intruder from the body. Inflammation also aids in the healing process and the repair of damaged tissue.

Chapter 3:

Planning and Prepping for Success

Planning and preparation are key to successfully implementing an anti-inflammatory diet. With a little bit of time and effort, you can set yourself up for success and make healthy eating a part of your daily routine.

Here are some tips for planning and preparing for success on an anti-inflammatory diet:

- Plan Your Meals: Spend some time every week organizing your meals. By doing this, you'll be able to stay on track and stop yourself from grabbing unhealthy foods when you're famished and pressed for time.

- Create a grocery list: Make a grocery list after you've planned your meals to ensure you have all the items. When you're at the store, follow your list to prevent making impulsive purchases.

- Prep Your Food: Spend some time cooking your meals so they are convenient to grab and go during the week. To do this, you might need to cut some veggies, prepare some grains, or make some snacks.

- Use Meal Prep Containers: It can be simple to portion out your meals for the week using meal prep containers. Use them to store prepared meals, snacks, and ingredients.

- Make use of leftovers:
- Don't throw out leftovers! Put them in your lunchbox the following day or use them as the foundation for a new dish.

- Cook in Bulk: Cooking in bulk can save you time during the week. Make a big batch of soup, chili, or stew and freeze portions for later.

- Keep Healthy Snacks on Hand: Ensure you have healthy snacks on hand so you're not tempted to reach for junk food when hunger strikes. Good options include fresh fruit, vegetables with hummus or guacamole, and nuts and seeds.

- Stay Organized: Keep your fridge and pantry organized so you can easily find what you need. This will also help you avoid buying duplicates of items you already have.

- Have a backup plan: Even with the best planning and preparation, things don't always go as planned. Have a backup plan so you're not left scrambling for a healthy meal option. This could be as simple as keeping some frozen veggies and a protein source on hand.

Planning your meals is one of the best strategies to guarantee success with an anti-inflammatory diet. This entails setting aside some time each week to prepare your meals and snacks. You may avoid impulse purchases and ensure you have everything you need to prepare wholesome meals throughout the week by doing so.

Another crucial stage in the planning and preparation process is preparing your food. Making healthy eating simple during the week can be accomplished by investing some time in chopping vegetables, cooking grains, and preparing snacks. You can portion up your meals and snacks in advance by using meal prep containers, making it easier for you to grab and go.

When it comes to preparing and planning, leftovers can sometimes come in quite handy. You can save time and cut down on food waste by using last night's meal for today's lunch. Another excellent way to save time during the week is to cook in bulk in quite handy. You can save time and cut down on food waste by using last night's meal for today's lunch. Another excellent way to save time during the week is to cook in bulk. Making a large quantity of soup, stew, or chili allows you to freeze individual servings for later use, ensuring you always have wholesome, delectable meals available.

Keeping healthy snacks on hand is another key aspect of planning and prepping. By stocking your fridge and pantry with fresh fruit, veggies, nuts, and seeds, you can easily satisfy your hunger and avoid reaching for unhealthy snacks when hunger strikes.

Finally, having a backup plan is always a good idea. Even with the best planning and preparation, things can go awry. Having a frozen veggie and protein source on hand can be a lifesaver when you're short on time or have unexpected guests.

In conclusion, preparation and planning are essential components of an effective anti-inflammatory diet. You can incorporate healthy eating into your daily routine by taking the time to plan your meals, make a grocery list, prepare your food, utilize meal prep containers, use leftovers, cook in bulk, keep healthy snacks on hand, stay organized, and have a backup plan. With a little bit of work, you can create healthy habits that will benefit you for years to come.

Chapter 4:

A 6-week meal-prep plan for anti-inflammatory

The 6-week meal prep plan for an anti-inflammatory diet consists of breakfast, lunch, dinner, and snack options that are rich in anti-inflammatory nutrients such as fruits, vegetables, whole grains, healthy fats, and lean proteins.

Each week's plan includes a variety of meals to provide essential nutrients and reduce inflammation in the body. The plan also emphasizes the use of cooking techniques that preserve the nutritional value of the food and minimize the use of processed ingredients.

The meal prep plan is designed to help individuals save time and money by planning and preparing meals in advance, making it easier to stick to an anti-inflammatory diet. It also helps individuals maintain a healthy weight, improve gut health, reduce the risk of chronic diseases, and improve overall well-being.

The plan is flexible and can be adjusted to meet individual needs and preferences. It also provides a guide for individuals to follow when grocery shopping and preparing meals to ensure they are consuming a balanced and nutritious diet.

Overall, the 6-week meal prep plan for an anti-inflammatory diet is an effective way to improve overall health and well-being by reducing inflammation in the body and promoting a balanced and nutritious diet.

Week 1:

Day	Breakfast	Lunch	Dinner	Snack
Mon	Avocado Toast with Tomatoes	Quinoa Salad with Vegetabl es	Grilled Chicken with Vegetabl es	Apple Slices with Almond Butter
Tues	Green Smoothie Bowl	Chickpe a and Spinach Curry	Baked Salmon with Asparag us	Carrots and Humm us
Wed	Sweet Potato Breakfast Bowl	Turkey and Veggie Wrap	Vegetabl e Stir-Fry	Mixed Nuts
Thu	Blueberry Chia Pudding	Salmon Salad	Turkey Meatball s with Zoodles	yogurt with berries
Fri	Greek Yogurt with Berries	Lentil Soup	Lentil Stew	Roasted chickpe as
Sat	Banana Pancakes	Sweet Potato and Black	Broiled Flank Steak with	Hard-boiled eggs with

		Bean Bowl	Roasted Veggies	Veggies
Sun	Spinach and Mushroom Omelette	Chicken Salad with Avocado	Shrimp and Quinoa Bowl	Celery with Peanut Butter

Week 2:

Day	Breakfast	Lunch	Dinner	Snack
Mon	Berry and Almond Butter Smoothie	Chicken Salad with Avocado	Shrimp and Quinoa Bowl	Roasted chickpeas
Tue	Sweet Potato Breakfast Bowl	Lentil Soup	Broiled Flank Steak with Roasted Veggies	Hard-boiled eggs with Veggies

Wed	Greek Yogurt with Berries	Turkey and Veggie Wrap	Grilled Chicken with Vegetables	Mixed Nuts
Thu	Banana pancakes	Sweet Potato and Black Bean Bowl	Vegetable Stir-Fry	yogurt with berries
Fri	Spinach and Mushroom Omelette	Quinoa Salad with Veggies	Lentil Stew	Apple Slices with Almond Butter
Sat	Chia Seed Pudding	Chickpea and Spinach Curry	Turkey Meatballs with Zoodles	Carrots and Hummus
Sun	Avocado Toast with Tomatoes	Salmon Salad	Baked Salmon with Asparagus	Celery with Peanut Butter

Week 3:

Day	Breakfast	Lunch	Dinner	Snack
Mon	Sweet Potato Breakfast Bowl	Quinoa and lentil salad	Turmeric Roasted Chicken Thighs with Cauliflower Rice	Sliced cucumber with hummus
Tue	Blueberry Chia Pudding	Grilled Chicken Salad with Spinach and Avocado	Baked salmon with roasted broccoli	Carrot Sticks with Almond Butter
Wed	Green Smoothie Bowl	Butternut Squash Soup with Turkey Meatbal	Vegetable Stir Fry with Brown Rice	Sliced Apple with Cashew Butter

		ls		
Thu	Apple Cinnamon Oatmeal	Grilled Vegetables with Chickpeas and Brown Rice	Lemon Garlic Shrimp with Zucchini Noodles	Cherry Tomatoes with Basil
Fri	Avocado Toast with Smoked Salmon	Turkey and Vegetable Skewers with Quinoa	Beef and Vegetable Stir Fry with Brown Rice	Roasted Almonds
Sat	Greek Yogurt Parfait with Berries and Granola	Tuna Salad Lettuce Wraps with Carrot Sticks	Grilled Mahi Mahi with Roasted Asparagus	Grapes
Sun	Mushroom and Spinach Frittata	Lentil Soup with Sliced Whole	Grilled Chicken with Sweet Potato	Baby Carrots with Hummus

		Grain Bread	Mash and Steamed Green Beans	

Week 4:

Day	Breakfast	Lunch	Dinner	Snack
Mon	Spinach and Feta Omelette	Quinoa and Vegetable Stuffed Bell Pepper	Slow Cooker Vegetable and Beef Stew	Raw Cashews
Tue	Coconut Flour Pancakes with Berries	Grilled Chicken Caesar Salad	Baked Cod with Roasted Brussels Sprouts	Sliced Apple with Almond Butter
Wed	Berry Smoothie with Chia Seeds	Roasted Vegetable and Chicken Salad	Pan-Seared Salmon with Cauliflo	Carrot Sticks with Hummus

			wer Mash	
Thu	Greek Yogurt with Berries and Walnuts	Turkey and Vegetabl e Chili	Grilled Flank Steak with Roasted Broccoli	Cherry Tomato es with Basil
Fri	Avocado Toast with Poached Egg	Tuna and Vegetabl e Salad	Chicken and Vegetab le Stir Fry with Brown Rice	Roasted Almond s
Sat	Breakfast Burrito with Sautéed Spinach and Feta	Grilled Shrimp Skewers with Quinoa	Slow Cooker Balsami c Chicken with Steame d Carrots	Grapes
Sun	Sweet Potato and Sausage	Lentil Soup with Sliced	Grilled Chicken with Sweet	Baby Carrots with Humm

	Breakfast Skillet	Whole Grain Bread	Potato Mash and Steamed Green Beans	us

Week 5:

Day	Breakfast	Lunch	Dinner	Snack
Mon	Green Smoothie Bowl	Quinoa Salad with Veggies	Baked Salmon with Asparagus	Carrot Sticks with Hummus
Tue	Breakfast Burrito Bowl	Veggie Wrap with Avocado Hummus	Slow Cooker Chili	Sliced Apple with Almond Butter
Wed	Yogurt with Berries and Granola	Chicken and Vegetable Stir-Fry	Roasted Vegetable and Quinoa Bowl	Celery with Nut Butter
Thu		Stuffed	Lentil	Dark

	Blueberry Chia Seed Pudding	Bell Pepper	Soup with Sweet Potato	Chocolate Square
Fri	Breakfast Salad	Tuna Salad Lettuce Wraps	Grilled Chicken with Roasted Veggies	Baked Sweet Potato Chips
Sat	Scrambled Eggs with Spinach	Tomato and Mozzarella Salad	Beef and Broccoli Stir-Fry	Greek Yogurt with Mixed Berries
Sun	Smoothie Bowl with Granola	Quinoa and Vegetable Bowl	Turkey Meatballs with Zucchini Noodles	Cucumber Slices with Hummus

Week 6:

Day	Breakfast	Lunch	Dinner	Snack
Mon	Chia Seed Pudding with Fruit	Tofu and Vegetable Stir-Fry	Spaghetti Squash with Meat Sauce	Sliced Cucumber with Guacamole
Tue	Breakfast Burrito Bowl	Egg Salad Lettuce Wraps	Grilled Salmon with Roasted Veggies	Apple Slices with Almond Butter
Wed	Yogurt with Berries and Nuts	Quinoa Salad with Roasted Veggies	Slow Cooker Chili	Carrot Sticks with Hummus
Thu	Green Smoothie Bowl	Chicken Caesar Salad	Beef and Broccoli Stir-Fry	Dark Chocolate Square
Fri	Breakfast Salad	Veggie Wrap	Roasted Vegetab	Baked Sweet

		with Avocado Hummus	le and Quinoa Bowl	Potato Chips
Sat	Scrambled Eggs with Spinach	Tuna Salad Lettuce Wraps	Grilled Chicken with Asparagus	Greek Yogurt with Mixed Berries
Sun	Smoothie Bowl with Granola	Lentil Soup with Sweet Potato	Turkey Meatballs with Zucchini Noodles	Celery with Nut Butter

Chapter 5:

Anti-Inflammatory Breakfast Ideas

Starting your day off with a nutritious, anti-inflammatory breakfast can set the tone for the rest of your day. In this chapter, we will explore some delicious breakfast ideas that are both easy to prepare and packed with anti-inflammatory ingredients.

- Smoothie Bowl: A variety of nutrients can be included in a smoothie bowl for a filling lunch. To ensure that you are getting a mix of vitamins and minerals, try to incorporate a variety of fruits and vegetables when constructing a smoothie bowl. Chia seeds or flaxseed can also provide a healthy serving of omega-3 fatty acids, which have anti-inflammatory effects, to your smoothie bowl. Several frozen berries, spinach, almond milk, and chia seeds can be blended together to make a healthy and energizing breakfast bowl. For extra crunch and taste, sprinkle some sliced almonds and fresh fruit on top.

- Avocado Toast: In recent years, avocado toast has grown in popularity as a breakfast item, and for good reason. Avocados are a fantastic source of fiber and good fats that can help you feel full and satisfied. Choose whole-grain bread instead of white bread, which can sometimes induce inflammation, to keep your avocado toast anti-inflammatory. Over a slice of whole-grain toast, mash up some ripe avocado. For a filling and healthy breakfast, add a sprinkle of red pepper flakes, a drizzle of olive oil, and a squeeze of fresh lemon juice on top.

- Veggie Omelet: Omelets are a flexible and simple breakfast choice, omelets can be tailored to your preferences. To ensure that you are getting a variety of nutrients, try to add a variety of colorful vegetables when preparing a veggie omelet. Great choices include bell peppers, onions, spinach, and mushrooms. Make an omelet by adding some sautéed spinach, bell peppers, and onions. Feta cheese can be included to add flavor and calcium.

- Quinoa Breakfast Bowl: Breakfast bowls can be made with quinoa because it is a versatile grain that works well in many different recipes. To get rid of any bitterness, properly rinse your quinoa before cooking. Sliced banana and almond butter can add a healthy serving of protein and good fats to your quinoa bowl. Prepare some quinoa, then add some almond butter, cinnamon, and banana slices on top. Because of its high protein and fiber content, quinoa will help you feel full and satisfied all morning long.

- Greek Yogurt Parfait: Choose plain Greek yogurt for your parfait rather than flavored yogurt, which might include a lot of extra sugar. Fresh berries and homemade granola can add a healthy serving of fiber and antioxidants to your parfait. For a tasty and filling breakfast, layer some plain Greek yogurt with fresh berries and granola. Greek yogurt has a lot of protein, and the addition of berries and oats increases its fiber and antioxidant content.

- Breakfast Tacos: Tacos aren't just for dinner! When making breakfast tacos, opt for whole wheat tortillas instead of white tortillas, which can cause inflammation in some individuals. Adding black beans and avocado to your tacos can provide a healthy dose of fiber and healthy fats. Fill a whole wheat tortilla with scrambled eggs, black beans, avocado, and salsa for a hearty and flavorful breakfast. The black beans provide a healthy dose of fiber and protein, while the avocado adds healthy fats and vitamins.

- Chia Pudding: Chia seeds are a great source of fiber and omega-3 fatty acids, which can help reduce inflammation in the body. When making chia pudding, be sure to let the mixture sit for at least 30 minutes to allow the chia seeds to absorb the liquid and thicken up. Adding fresh fruit and nuts to your chia pudding can provide added flavor and texture. Mix some chia seeds, almond milk, vanilla extract, and honey for a simple and nutritious breakfast pudding. Top with some fresh fruit and sliced almonds for added flavor and crunch.

- Turmeric Scrambled Eggs: Turmeric is a powerful anti-inflammatory spice that can be added to scrambled eggs for a flavorful and nutritious breakfast. Simply whisk turmeric into your eggs before cooking, and add in some vegetables like spinach or bell peppers for added nutrition.

- Breakfast Burrito Bowl: For a hearty and satisfying breakfast, consider making a breakfast burrito bowl. Start with a base of brown rice or quinoa, and add scrambled eggs, black beans, avocado, and salsa for a flavorful and nutritious meal.

- Sweet Potato Toast: Sweet potatoes are a nutritious and anti-inflammatory alternative to traditional toast. Slice a sweet potato into thin rounds and toast them in the toaster or under the broiler. Top with avocado smoked salmon, or nut butter for a filling and satisfying breakfast.

- Green Smoothie: Starting your day with a green smoothie is a great way to get in a variety of nutrients and antioxidants. Blend spinach, kale, cucumber, celery, and apple for a refreshing and anti-inflammatory smoothie.

- Overnight Oats: Overnight oats are a convenient and nutritious breakfast option that can be customized to your liking. Mix rolled oats, almond milk, chia seeds, and your favorite toppings like nuts, seeds, and berries. Let the mixture sit in the refrigerator overnight, and enjoy it in the morning for a filling and nutritious meal.

- Tofu Scramble: For a plant-based and anti-inflammatory breakfast option, consider making a tofu scramble. Crumble firm tofu into a pan and cook with vegetables like spinach, bell peppers, and mushrooms. Season with turmeric, garlic, and nutritional yeast for added flavor.

- Homemade Breakfast Bars: Store-bought breakfast bars can be high in added sugars and processed ingredients. Instead, consider making your breakfast bars using oats, nuts, seeds, and dried fruit. This way, you can control the ingredients and ensure that your breakfast is anti-inflammatory and nutritious.

In conclusion, there are plenty of delicious and nutritious anti-inflammatory breakfast options to choose from. Whether you prefer a smoothie bowl, avocado toast, veggie omelet, quinoa breakfast bowl, Greek yogurt parfait, breakfast tacos, chia pudding, and so on, these meals will help you start your day off on the right foot. By incorporating these breakfast ideas into your daily routine, you can support your body's natural anti-inflammatory processes and promote overall health and wellness.

Chapter 6:

Anti-Inflammatory Lunch Ideas

Lunch is an important meal that provides the energy and nutrients needed to power through the rest of the day. When following an anti-inflammatory diet, it's important to choose nutrient-dense foods that are high in antioxidants and anti-inflammatory compounds. Here are some ideas for delicious and nutritious anti-inflammatory lunch options:

- Barbecued Chicken and Vegetable Plate of mixed greens: In addition to being high in nutrients that are anti-inflammatory, grilled chicken and vegetables are an excellent source of protein and fiber. Grilled chicken, bell peppers, zucchini, and onions on a bed of mixed greens are topped with a homemade vinaigrette made with olive oil, lemon juice, and garlic.

- Quinoa and Vegetable Bowl: Quinoa is a whole grain with a lot of protein and a lot of compounds that fight inflammation. For a filling and nutritious lunch, combine cooked quinoa, roasted sweet potatoes, broccoli, and cauliflower, and drizzle with a creamy avocado dressing.

- Lentil Soup: Lentils are full of anti-inflammatory compounds and are an excellent source of plant-based protein. Make a generous lentil soup by stewing lentils with vegetables like carrots, celery, and onions, and adding calming flavors like turmeric and cumin.

- Wraps with lettuce and tuna: Omega-3 fatty acids, which have anti-inflammatory properties, can be found in abundance in tuna. For a light and healthy lunch, combine diced celery, red onion, and avocado with canned tuna and wrap it in lettuce.

- Curry with Chickpeas and Vegetables: In addition to being a great source of protein and fiber, chickpeas contain a lot of anti-inflammatory compounds. By simmering chickpeas, cauliflower, spinach, and tomato in anti-inflammatory spices like ginger, turmeric, and cinnamon, you can make a flavorful chickpea and vegetable curry.

- Zucchini Noodle Pasta: Zucchini noodles are an extraordinary low-carb option in contrast to customary pasta, and are likewise wealthy in mitigating compounds. For a filling and nutritious lunch, spiralize zucchini into noodles, sauté it with garlic and cherry tomatoes, and top it with grilled chicken or shrimp.

- Toast with Sardine and Avocado: Sardines are a great source of omega-3 fatty acids and contain a lot of compounds that fight inflammation. For a quick and healthy lunch option, spread mashed avocado on the whole-grain toast. Add sardines and a squeeze of lemon on top.

- Salmon and asparagus roasted: Salmon is an excellent source of anti-inflammatory nutrients and omega-3 fatty acids. Cook salmon and asparagus with garlic and lemon for a straightforward and tasty lunch.

- Chicken and Vegetable Sautéed food: A quick and simple way to include a variety of vegetables in your diet is through stir-fry. Season chicken with anti-inflammatory spices like turmeric and ginger while sautéing broccoli, bell peppers, carrots, and onions.

- Wrap with Hummus and Turkey: Turkey is full of nutrients that fight inflammation and is a low-calorie source of protein. For a healthy and filling lunch, spread hummus on a whole-grain wrap and top it with sliced turkey, spinach, and roasted red peppers.

- Stir-Fry with Vegetables and Lentil: Lentils are full of anti-inflammatory compounds and are an excellent source of plant-based protein. Season lentils with anti-inflammatory spices like cumin and coriander while sautéing vegetables like zucchini, mushrooms, and onions.

- Burger with Grilled Portobello Mushrooms: Portobello mushrooms are a good source of protein for vegetarians and contain a lot of nutrients that fight inflammation. For a delicious and nutritious lunch, grill portobello mushrooms and serve them on a whole-grain bun with avocado and sliced tomatoes.

- Burrito Bowl with Sweet Potatoes and Black Beans: In addition to being a great source of complex carbohydrates and anti-inflammatory nutrients, sweet potatoes are also delicious. For a filling and nutritious lunch bowl, combine avocado, brown rice, black beans, and roasted sweet potatoes.

- Shrimp and vegetable sticks: Shrimp is a lean wellspring of protein and is likewise wealthy in mitigating compounds. Stick shrimp with vegetables like chime peppers, onions, and cherry tomatoes, and barbecue or dish for a tasty and nutritious lunch.

In conclusion, incorporating anti-inflammatory foods into your lunch can provide numerous health benefits, including reducing inflammation in the body, improving gut health, and supporting a healthy immune system. The lunch ideas provided in this chapter are not only delicious but also easy to prepare and can be customized to suit your preferences and dietary needs. By choosing whole, nutrient-dense foods and incorporating anti-inflammatory herbs and spices, you can create a balanced and satisfying lunch that supports your overall health and well-being. Additionally, planning and prepping your lunches in advance can help you stay on track with your anti-inflammatory diet and save time and money in the long run. So, whether you're at home, at work, or on the go, these anti-inflammatory lunch ideas are a great way to fuel your body and keep inflammation at bay.

Chapter 7:

Anti-Inflammatory Dinner Ideas
Dinner is an important meal when it comes to an anti-inflammatory diet for several reasons. Firstly, the foods we eat at dinner can impact our sleep quality and overall recovery, which plays a crucial role in managing inflammation. Secondly, it's an opportunity to fuel our body with nutrient-dense, anti-inflammatory ingredients that can help reduce inflammation and promote overall health. Here are some ideas for delicious and nutritious anti-inflammatory dinner options:

- Heated Salmon with Broiled Vegetables: Omega-3 fatty acids, which have anti-inflammatory properties, are abundant in salmon. For a balanced meal, combine it with roasted vegetables like carrots, broccoli, and asparagus.

- Peppers with Quinoa and Vegetable Stuffing: Quinoa is a gluten-free, anti-inflammatory grain with a lot of protein. For a filling and nutritious meal, stuff bell peppers with quinoa, sautéed vegetables, and herbs.
- Turkey Stew: A flavorful and filling chili can be made with ground turkey, a protein that is low in calories and high in protein. For additional health benefits, add anti-inflammatory ingredients like beans, tomatoes, and chili powder.
- Chicken and Vegetables Roasted: Combining roasted vegetables like sweet potatoes, Brussels sprouts, and carrots with roasted chicken is an easy way to make a classic dinner even healthier.
- Vegetable Curry: Ginger, turmeric, and garlic are common anti-inflammatory ingredients in curry dishes. For a nutritious and flavorful

dinner, use a variety of vegetables like cauliflower, spinach, and eggplant.

- Lenten Soup: Lentils are an incredible wellspring of plant-based protein and are likewise calming. Combine them with vegetables like kale, carrots, and celery to make a hearty and filling soup.
- Barbecued tofu and vegetable sticks: Tofu is a protein derived from plants that are loaded with anti-inflammatory substances. For a flavorful and nutritious dinner option, skewer it with a variety of vegetables, like bell peppers, onions, and mushrooms.
- Avocado Salsa and Grilled Salmon: A delicious and anti-inflammatory dinner option is grilled salmon with fresh avocado salsa on top. Avocado is wealthy in monounsaturated fats, which have been shown to have calming properties.

- Chickpea and vegetable sautés: chickpeas contain anti-inflammatory properties and are an excellent source of plant-based protein. For a flavorful and nutritious dinner, combine them with broccoli, bell peppers, onions, and garlic in a vegetable stir-fry.
- Rice and Cauliflower Bowl: In addition to being anti-inflammatory, cauliflower rice is a low-carb, gluten-free alternative to regular rice. For a satisfying and nutritious dinner option, top it with grilled chicken, roasted vegetables, and a drizzle of tahini sauce.
- Zucchini Noodles with Turkey Meatballs: Zoodles, or zucchini noodles, are a low-carb, anti-inflammatory alternative to conventional pasta. Match them with handcrafted turkey meatballs and a pureed tomato dish made with mitigating spices and flavors like basil, oregano, and turmeric.

- Sweet Potato Stuffed: For a filling and nutritious dinner option, sweet potatoes, a nutrient-dense, and anti-inflammatory vegetable, can be stuffed with black beans, quinoa, and avocado.
- Curry with Vegetables and Lentils: For a flavorful and anti-inflammatory curry, vegetables and lentils are a great combination. For additional health benefits, include anti-inflammatory herbs and spices like ginger, turmeric, and cumin.
- Caesar Salad with Grilled Chicken: Barbecued chicken matched with a natively constructed Caesar dressing made with mitigating fixings like garlic, Dijon mustard, and lemon juice is a delightful and sound supper choice.

Incorporating these anti-inflammatory dinner ideas into your meal planning can provide numerous health benefits and help reduce inflammation in the body. Additionally, by choosing whole, nutrient-dense ingredients and incorporating anti-inflammatory herbs and spices, you can create delicious and satisfying meals that support your overall health and well-being.

Chapter 8:

Anti-Inflammatory Snack Ideas
Snacks can play an important role in an anti-inflammatory diet by providing a way to incorporate nutrient-dense foods into your diet between meals. Anti-inflammatory snacks can help stabilize blood sugar levels, provide sustained energy, and reduce inflammation in the body.

- Cut cucumbers with hummus: Cucumbers are a hydrating and refreshing snack because they are low in calories and high in water. For a filling and nutritious snack, pair them with hummus, which is made with chickpeas, tahini, olive oil, and other anti-inflammatory ingredients.
- Slices of apple with almond butter: Almond butter is a nutrient-dense and anti-inflammatory source of healthy fats, and apples are an excellent

source of fiber and antioxidants. This snack is a great mid-afternoon pick-me-up because it is delicious and filling.

- Kale Chips: By roasting it in the oven, you can turn kale, a nutrient-dense, and anti-inflammatory vegetable, into a delicious and crispy snack. Simply toss the kale with your preferred herbs and spices and olive oil before baking at a low temperature until crispy.
- Yogurt from Greece with Berries: Probiotics, which support a healthy gut microbiome and reduce inflammation, can be found in Greek yogurt, making it an excellent source of protein. For a tasty and healthy snack, combine it with berries like blueberries or strawberries that are high in antioxidants.
- Chickpeas roasted: chickpeas contain anti-inflammatory properties and are an excellent source of plant-based protein. Broil them with your favorite

spices and flavors for a crunchy and fulfilling nibble.

- A Toast of Avocado: Monounsaturated fats, which have been shown to reduce inflammation, can be found in abundance in avocados. Match it with whole-wheat toast and a sprinkle of calming spices and flavors like turmeric and dark pepper for a fantastic and nutritious tidbit.
- Trail Mix: Healthy fats, fiber, and antioxidants can all be found in abundance in a homemade trail mix made with nuts, seeds, and dried fruit. In order to keep it as anti-inflammatory as possible, look for options that are unsweetened and unseasoned.
- Sticks of carrot with guacamole: Guacamole is made with anti-inflammatory ingredients like avocados, lime juice, and cilantro, and carrots are high in fiber and

antioxidants. Snacks made with this combination are filling and delicious.

- Tomatoes with balsamic vinegar and cherries: Cherry tomatoes are a decent wellspring of L-ascorbic acid and lycopene, which are the two cell reinforcements that can assist with diminishing irritation. For a snack with a sweet and sour flavor, drizzle them with balsamic vinegar.

- Edamame: Edamame is full of anti-inflammatory nutrients like folate, vitamin C, and fiber, making it an excellent source of plant-based protein. Sea salt can be added to edamame by simply steaming or boiling it.

- Chia Seed Pudding: Chia seeds are wealthy in fiber, omega-3 unsaturated fats, and cell reinforcements, which can assist with decreasing irritation in the body. For a tasty and healthy snack, combine chia seeds, your preferred non-dairy milk, and a dash of honey or maple syrup.

- Cooked Beet Chips: Beets are a supplement, a thick root vegetable that is wealthy in calming compounds like betalains and fiber. Daintily cut beets and roast them in the broiler until fresh for a solid and heavenly bite.
- Chocolate: Dark, dusky chocolate is wealthy in cell reinforcements and flavonols, which can assist with lessening aggravation in the body. For maximum anti-inflammatory benefits, select high-quality dark chocolate with a cocoa content of at least 70%.
- Corn with Turmeric: For a tasty and nutritious snack, you can add turmeric to popcorn, which is a potent anti-inflammatory spice. For a flavorful and healthy snack, simply sprinkle popcorn with turmeric and a pinch of sea salt.

Incorporating these anti-inflammatory snack ideas into your daily routine can help support your overall health and well-being. By choosing whole, nutrient-dense ingredients and avoiding processed and high-sugar options, you can help reduce inflammation in the body and feel your best.

Chapter 9:

Anti-Inflammatory Dessert Ideas
When most people think of dessert, they often envision sugary, calorie-dense treats that aren't particularly healthy. However, with a little creativity, it's possible to enjoy delicious desserts that are both satisfying and anti-inflammatory.

When choosing anti-inflammatory desserts, it's important to focus on whole foods that are nutrient-dense and low in added sugars. This includes fruits, nuts, seeds, and healthy fats like avocado and coconut oil. Some examples of anti-inflammatory desserts include:

- Fruit salad with a drizzle of honey and chopped nuts
- Homemade chia seed pudding with berries and almond butter
- Baked apples with cinnamon and a sprinkle of walnuts

- Dark chocolate-covered strawberries
- Frozen banana "ice cream" with cocoa powder and almond milk
- Avocado chocolate mousse made with cacao powder and coconut milk
- Almond butter energy bites made with oats, dates, and cinnamon
- Berry crumbles made with oats, almond flour, and coconut oil

By making healthy swaps and using wholesome ingredients, it's possible to enjoy desserts that are both delicious and anti-inflammatory. These desserts can be a great way to satisfy your sweet tooth while still supporting your overall health and well-being.

Here are some additional tips for making anti-inflammatory desserts:

- Select fruits with a lot of antioxidants: Due to their abundance of antioxidants and anti-inflammatory compounds, berries, cherries, and pomegranates are excellent choices for anti-inflammatory desserts. They are delicious in fruit salads, smoothies, and oatmeal toppings.

- Use good fats: Avocado, nuts, and seeds, all of which contain healthy fats, can assist in reducing body inflammation. Energy bites, nut butter cups, and even a creamy chocolate mousse are all possible uses for them.
- Switch to natural sweeteners for refined sugar: Natural sweeteners like honey, maple syrup, or dates can be used in place of refined sugar in desserts. These sugars are lower on the glycemic index and won't cause similar spikes in that frame of mind as refined sugar.
- Try different spices: Many flavors have calming properties and can add flavor to your treats without adding sugar. Ginger, turmeric, and cinnamon are all excellent choices.

Remember, desserts should still be enjoyed in moderation, even if they're made with healthier ingredients. By incorporating anti-inflammatory desserts into your diet in moderation, you can satisfy your sweet tooth while still supporting your overall health and well-being.

Chapter 10:

Anti-Inflammatory Drinks and Beverages When it comes to staying hydrated on an anti-inflammatory diet, it's important to choose beverages that are low in sugar and high in antioxidants. Here are some examples of anti-inflammatory drinks and beverages:

- Green tea: catechins, which are antioxidants with anti-inflammatory properties, are abundant in green tea. It also has caffeine, which can naturally give you more energy.
- Latte with ginger: Curcumin, a substance found in spice turmeric, has potent anti-inflammatory properties. Warm milk can be combined with turmeric, cinnamon, ginger, and honey to make a turmeric latte.
- Lemon juice and water: Drinking lemon water is an easy way to stay hydrated and get your daily dose of

vitamin C, which has anti-inflammatory properties.

- Juice fraîche: A refreshing way to get a variety of anti-inflammatory nutrients is to drink juice made from fruits and vegetables like carrots, beets, and oranges that have been freshly squeezed.
- Kombucha: Probiotics, found in fermented teas like kombucha, can support a healthy gut microbiome. Ginger and turmeric, two anti-inflammatory herbs, are also present in some brands of kombucha.
- Gold milk: Brilliant milk is a customary Indian drink made with turmeric, ginger, and warm milk. It has a lot of compounds that are good for inflammation, so drinking it before bed can be relaxing.
- Matcha latte: Matcha tea is high in cancer prevention agents called catechins, which have calming

properties. Caffeine in it can also help increase alertness and concentration.

- Hibiscus tea is high in cancer prevention agents called anthocyanins, which have calming properties. It has also been shown to help lower cholesterol levels and blood pressure.
- Ginger tea: Ginger has anti-inflammatory properties thanks to compounds known as gingerols. Ginger tea is a warming and reassuring beverage that can assist in calming an upset stomach.
- Fruit smoothie: anthocyanins—antioxidants found in berries like strawberries, blueberries, and raspberries—have anti-inflammatory properties. Mix frozen berries with almond milk or yogurt for a reviving and nourishing pressed smoothie.
- Juice of watermelons: Lycopene, an antioxidant with anti-inflammatory

properties, is abundant in watermelons. Mix pieces of watermelon with lime juice and mint for a refreshing and hydrating drink.

Remember to choose drinks that are low in added sugars and artificial sweeteners, which can be pro-inflammatory. By incorporating a variety of these anti-inflammatory drinks and beverages into your diet, you can support your body's natural inflammatory response and promote overall health and well-being.

Chapter 11:

Cooking Techniques for an Anti-Inflammatory Diet

Cooking techniques play an important role in an anti-inflammatory diet. Certain cooking methods can help preserve the anti-inflammatory properties of the foods we eat, while others can increase inflammation. In this chapter, we will explore some of the best cooking techniques for an anti-inflammatory diet.

- Steaming: Vegetables can be preserved by steaming, a gentle cooking method that preserves their nutrients and anti-inflammatory compounds. Additionally, steaming helps preserve the food's natural flavors and textures without adding any additional fats or oils.
- Stir-frying: Vegetables and lean proteins can be cooked in a healthy

and quick manner by stir-frying. With just a little oil and preparing the food rapidly over high intensity, you can safeguard the supplements and mitigate the intensities in the food.

- Grilling: Cooking vegetables, fish, and other lean proteins on the grill is an excellent method. Just make sure to marinate your proteins first to help cut down on harmful, potentially inflammatory compounds like polycyclic aromatic hydrocarbons (PAHs) and heterocyclic amines (HCAs).

- Roasting: Broiling is a dry-intensity cooking strategy that can assist with drawing out the normal pleasantness and kinds of vegetables. Additionally, roasting aids in the preservation of the food's nutrients and anti-inflammatory compounds.

- Boiling: Bubbling is a straightforward and sound method for cooking vegetables and grains. Simply make certain to utilize an insignificant measure of water and abstain from overcooking, which can cause the deficiency of supplements.

- Cooking slowly: Slow cooking is a delicate and tasty method for cooking lean proteins like chicken and hamburgers. Slow cooking likewise assists with separating hard filaments in meats, making them more delicate and simple to process.
- Poaching: Cooking food in a small amount of liquid, like broth or water, is called poaching. In addition to adding flavor, this method of gentle cooking can assist in the preservation of the food's nutrients and anti-inflammatory compounds.
- Broiling: Searing is a dry-intensity cooking technique that can be utilized to rapidly cook lean proteins and vegetables. Be careful not to overcook or burn the food because doing so can make inflammation worse, but this

method can help preserve the food's nutrients and anti-inflammatory compounds.

- Sautéing: The fast cooking of food in a small amount of oil over high heat is known as sautéing. This strategy can be utilized to cook vegetables, lean proteins, and entire grains. For added flavor and health benefits, use olive oil or coconut oil and anti-inflammatory spices like ginger or turmeric.
- Juicing and blending: Mixing and squeezing can be an incredible method for integrating more calming products of the soil into your eating routine. By mixing or pressing your foods grown from the ground, you can make delectable and nutritious beverages that are wealthy in cell reinforcements and other mitigating compounds.

By using these cooking techniques, you can help support your body's natural inflammatory response and promote overall health and well-being. Remember to also choose healthy, anti-inflammatory ingredients and avoid processed and fried foods as much as possible.

Chapter 12:

Building an Anti-Inflammatory Pantry

Building an anti-inflammatory pantry is an essential step towards success on an anti-inflammatory diet. By having the right ingredients on hand, you can easily prepare healthy and delicious meals that support your body's natural inflammatory response. Here are some key components of an anti-inflammatory pantry:

- Whole Cereals: Entire grains are a brilliant wellspring of fiber, which can assist with advancing solid assimilation and diminish aggravation. Additionally, they contain anti-inflammatory vitamins and minerals like selenium, magnesium, and B vitamins. Look for whole grain options like brown rice, quinoa, whole wheat pasta, and whole grain bread when shopping for whole grains.

- Seeds and nuts: Healthy fats, which can support heart health and reduce inflammation, are abundant in nuts and seeds. Additionally, they contain protein, dietary fiber, and other nutrients that can aid in maintaining a full and satisfied stomach. Almonds, walnuts, chia seeds, flaxseeds, and pumpkin seeds are excellent choices.
- Legumes: A great source of plant-based protein, fiber, and other nutrients that can help reduce inflammation are lentils, chickpeas, and black beans. They can also be used in a wide range of dishes, including dips, salads, stews, and soups.
- Sound Fats: Sound fats like extra-virgin olive oil, coconut oil, and avocado oil can assist with decreasing aggravation and supporting heart well-being. They can also enhance the flavor and richness of your meals and serve as an excellent energy source.

- Spices and Flavors: Spices and herbs are a great way to flavor food and improve your health. Anti-inflammatory compounds in turmeric, ginger, garlic, and cinnamon, among other herbs and spices, can assist in reducing body inflammation.
- Fresh Fruit: Fiber, vitamins, and minerals can all be found in abundance in fresh fruits and vegetables, which can also assist in reducing body inflammation. Try to get a wide range of colors so you can get a wide range of nutrients.
- Broth with Low Sodium: Low-sodium stock can be utilized as a base for soups and stews and can add flavor and supplements without adding an overabundance of sodium. Look for options that don't contain any artificial ingredients or preservatives.

By building an anti-inflammatory pantry, you'll be able to easily create healthy and delicious meals that support your body's natural inflammatory response. Remember to also choose high-quality, organic ingredients as much as possible, and to avoid processed and fried foods. With a little planning and preparation, you'll be on your way to a healthier, more vibrant life!

Chapter 13:

Overcoming Obstacles to Meal Prep

Meal prepping can be an effective way to stick to an anti-inflammatory diet, but it can also come with its own set of challenges. In this chapter, we will discuss some of the common obstacles that people face when trying to meal prep for an anti-inflammatory diet and provide some strategies to overcome them.

- Limitations on time: Finding the time to meal prep is one of the biggest obstacles that people face. It can be hard to make time for food preparation and grocery shopping when you have a full schedule. Set aside a specific time each week to plan and prepare your meals to overcome this obstacle. This will assist you with focusing on feast prep and guarantee that you have the opportunity to make it happen.

- Lack of enthusiasm: Lack of inspiration is another common obstacle to meal preparation. If you're used to eating pre-packaged or processed foods, it can be hard to come up with new and exciting meal ideas. To defeat this test, have a go at perusing mitigating recipes online, joining a dinner prep bunch, or exploring different avenues regarding new fixings and cooking methods.
- Cost: Eating a sound, mitigating diet can once in a while be more costly than an eating routine that incorporates handled and pre-bundled food varieties. For people who are on a tight budget, this could be a significant obstacle. To conquer this test, think about purchasing fixings in bulk, buying frozen produce, and consolidating more affordable sources of protein like beans and lentils.
- Lack of cooking supplies: Healthy cooking can sometimes necessitate

specialized kitchen tools that you might not have on hand. To defeat this test, begin with straightforward, fundamental feasts that require negligible hardware and step by step assemble your assortment of kitchen apparatuses over the long haul.

- Trouble staying on track: Finally, adhering to the plan is one of the biggest roadblocks to successful meal prep. Life can be erratic, and you very well may be trying to adhere to a meal prep plan when surprising occasions emerge. Be adaptable and willing to make any necessary adjustments to your meal plan to overcome this obstacle. Keep solid, calming snacks available for those times when you can't adhere to your arrangement, and don't be too unforgiving with yourself in the event that things don't go as expected.

By recognizing and overcoming these common obstacles to meal prep, you can make it easier to stick to an anti-inflammatory diet and enjoy the many benefits that come with it.

In conclusion, adopting an anti-inflammatory diet can be a powerful tool in improving your overall health and well-being. The science behind inflammation and the role of diet in its management is well established, and the benefits of a balanced, nutrient-dense diet are clear.

With the tips, recipes, and strategies provided in this book, you can begin to make small but impactful changes to your eating habits. By incorporating more whole, unprocessed foods and limiting inflammatory ingredients, you can support your body's natural healing processes and reduce your risk of chronic diseases.

Meal prepping is an essential tool in making the switch to an anti-inflammatory diet. By planning and preparing your meals ahead of time, you can ensure that you always have healthy, nourishing options on hand, even on busy days.

Remember, making changes to your diet and lifestyle takes time and effort, but the results are well worth it. By following the guidance in this book and listening to your body's needs, you can take control of your health and live a happier, more vibrant life.

www.ingramcontent.com/pod-product-compliance
Lightning Source LLC
Chambersburg PA
CBHW070445220526
45466CB00004B/1771